No One Told Me

What Every Family Needs to Know About Mental Illness in America

Kimberly A. Bowman

KI Productions

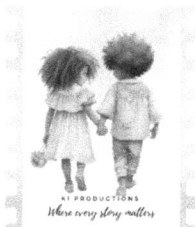

KI PRODUCTIONS
Where every story matters

DEDICATION

*I want to dedicate this book to all the moms,
dads, and caregivers who have ever walked this
journey. You are stronger than you think you are
and you have never walked alone. If you are still
on the path, I pray you feel more empowered,
equipped, and focused to continue the journey.*

I also dedicate this book to my sons:

*I love you both more than words can express. I've
prayed for you since the day you were born and I
have continued every day since. I know that God
has a grip on you and He isn't letting go.*

tament to the real world struggles for both the afflicted and the caregiver. You will no longer feel alone after reading Kim's book. ~ Alison Thompson, Professional Paralegal

Contents

FOREWORD

Since the dawn of the deinstitutionalization movement more than 60 years ago, our politicians and our communities have failed to provide adequate community support systems for persons afflicted with serious mental illness. Consequently, many people have ended up in the streets, and our jails and prisons have replaced psychiatric hospitals as the places of involuntary confinement and "humane" treatment.

Thanks to ground-breaking research conducted by the MacArthur Foundation we now know that persons with mental illness are no more violent than the general population, yet they continue to be locked up for minor, quality-of-life offenses, like shoplifting and drug possession. Many jurisdictions have created well-intentioned mental health units in their jails and mental health diversion programs in their courts, but they are working against long odds. Putting aside that penal institutions are inherently not places to get well, defendants are released, often abruptly, without support of any kind. No money, no job, no housing, no connection to treatment, not even a valid ID. Even in the best case scenario, they are released to a system of woefully underfunded community-based services. Is it any wonder we have created a revolving door of relapse, offending, arrest, and detention?

As a public defender specializing in representation of persons with mental illness for over twenty years, I have dealt with the consequences of this broken system. Perhaps that's why Kimberly Bowman reached out to me for advice in her ongoing efforts to extract her son from the criminal justice system and get appropriate mental health services in place for him. Over the course of many phone conversations, I'm certain I learned as much from her as she did from me. She has a unique perspective gleaned from years of tracking her son's encounters with the criminal justice system and advocating for him to be treated fairly and humanely. Constantly exhorting corrections officers, prosecutors, defense attorneys, and mental health workers to do the right thing so that her son could be released to appropriate mental health services required persistence, savvy, determination, a very stubborn faith, and, of course, a mother's love.

In *No One Told Me*, she does us a great favor by sharing all the lessons that she had to learn for herself the hard way. Unfortunately, what she has to say paints a pretty bleak picture: the mental health system is broken and the criminal justice system is a poor substitute for it. However, she doesn't just leave us hanging in a cloud of gloom and doom. She offers solid advice for how we can best navigate the systems as they are and increase the odds in favor of sustained recovery for our loved ones.

She will have much more to say in her forthcoming full-length book. She will share much more about her son's saga and her encounters with the mental health and criminal justice systems that will shed light on the criminalization of mental illness and point to a way forward and out of the morass.

Dave Norman

Retired Public Defender Mental Health Specialist

Introduction

The call came late—one of those nights when your heart knows before your ears do that everything is about to change.

My son was in crisis again, and I found myself standing in the middle of a system that felt more like a maze than a lifeline. I was told to wait. To call back. To "let the process work." But what no one told me was that the process itself was broken—or maybe, that it never really existed at all.

No one told me this would be so hard. No one told me that when your child's illness becomes visible, your world can collapse under the weight of paperwork, policies, and people who say they care but have no power to act. No one told me that love, as fierce as it is, cannot always navigate a system that was never designed for healing.

When mental illness enters a family, it doesn't knock—it bursts through the door and re-arranges everything. It challenges your faith, tests your marriage, drains your savings, and isolates you from the very community you need most. And while you're trying to hold your loved one together, you realize you have to hold the system accountable, too.

This book was born out of those sleepless nights, the endless phone calls, and the quiet grief that comes when you realize you're fighting an invisible war. It's also born out of hope—a fierce, stubborn belief that families can do more than survive; we can change the story.

No One Told Me is not a manual written from theory. It's a lived map. It's the hard lessons I learned the hardest way possible, shared so others might find a clearer path. In these pages, you'll learn what no one told me: how the system actually works, what rights you and your loved ones really have, how to speak the language of care and advocacy, and how to keep your hope alive when the waiting feels endless.

This is for every parent, sibling, spouse, or friend who has ever asked, Why didn't anyone tell me? You're not alone. There is a way through this. And once we begin to see the system for what it truly is, we can begin the work of rebuilding what it was always meant to be—human.

Preface

When I began writing this book, I didn't set out to become an expert on mental health systems, policy, or advocacy. I was simply a mother trying to keep her child safe. What I learned along the way—through sleepless nights, closed doors, and countless "no one told me" moments—is that the greatest crisis in mental health isn't just the illness itself. It's the silence that surrounds it.

Families are thrown into a world they don't understand, where help is fragmented and hope feels conditional. One agency handles housing, another manages treatment, and still another determines eligibility for care—none of them working together, all of them operating on timelines that don't match human urgency. The system is often described as "broken," but I've come to believe something harder and truer: we don't have a system. We have disconnected parts trying to function as a whole.

This book isn't meant to shame professionals or point fingers. It's meant to tell the truth—to name what families live through when a loved one's illness collides with institutions that were never designed for healing. It's also meant to give language, context, and courage to those who are still searching for answers.

Each lesson in this book grew from lived experience—mine, and that of countless parents, siblings, and caregivers who have walked this same uneven ground. Together, we are piecing together something that has been missing for too long: a map.

I also want you to know this: I am a woman of faith. My faith has been my anchor through every storm, my grounding when fear felt too heavy to carry. You'll see quiet glimpses of that faith in these pages—not in sermons, but in Scripture. They're meant as moments of breath. You can linger there, pray there, or simply rest there. Whether faith is a part of your journey or not, you are welcome here. This book was written for all who love someone living with mental illness and for anyone who believes we can build something better together.

My hope is that *No One Told Me* helps you feel less alone, more informed, and more empowered to ask hard questions. Because change doesn't begin in systems—it begins in stories. It begins when one voice dares to say, This isn't working, and another echoes, You're right.

May this little book remind you that knowledge is power, truth is advocacy, and hope is still possible—even here.

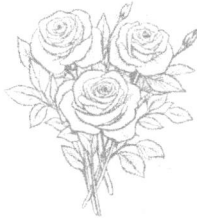

And we know that in all things God works for the good of those who love him, who have been called according to his purpose.

Romans 8:28

LESSON 1
NO ONE TOLD ME THE SYSTEM WASN'T DESIGNED FOR HEALING

(Spoiler: It's not broken. We never built it with intention to heal in the first place.)

I remember the exact moment the illusion shattered.

For years, I fought like hell—believing I was working *within* a flawed but ultimately well-meaning system. I thought if I just learned and followed the system better, persisted long enough, advocated fiercely enough, I could unlock the path to healing for my son. I believed that the services existed somewhere out there: the long-term treatment plans, compassionate providers, housing supports, coordinated care teams. I believed in the myth that the "system" was in place and it would be our safety net.

But that belief died slowly.

Courtroom by courtroom.

Crisis by crisis.

Discharge by discharge.

It died the day the hospital released my son with no safety plan.

When law enforcement showed up with hand-cuffs instead of help.

When the ER held him overnight only to say, "He doesn't meet the criteria."

When he slept in a jail cells for months because there was nowhere else for him to go.

It died the day I realized the waiting list for community mental health services was longer than the time he could stay stable without them.

That's when it hit me like a gut punch:

This wasn't a system that was failing to work.

This *was* how it worked.

And it was never meant to work for us.

———

We do not have a broken system. We have a disconnected, disjointed, and dysfunctional patchwork of institutions that manage crises without ever preventing them. It is reactive, not proactive. Bureaucratic, not human-centered. It is less a system of care and more a maze of survival. The farther I went, the more I understood—families like mine weren't falling through cracks; we were walking straight into gaps that were deliberately never filled.

And the most devastating part?

No one tells you this at the beginning.

You aren't handed a guidebook. You aren't told what to expect. You find out through the bruises and the silence. Through the 3 a.m. hospital discharges, the police calls, the missing persons reports. Through the weariness that sets in when your desperate calls for help are met with rules, waitlists, and warnings.

The Criminalization of Mental Illness

There is a deeply disturbing truth that haunts every parent, caregiver, or loved one walking this road: in America, the first time many people receive any kind of mental health intervention is in the back of a police car—or behind bars.

In America today, individuals with untreated mental illness are far more likely to be incarcerated than hospitalized. After the deinstitutionalization movement of the 1960s and '70s—when psychiatric hospitals were closed en masse—there was a promise: that robust, well-funded community mental health services would rise to take their place. That promise was broken. What followed instead was a vacuum, into which jails, shelters, and emergency rooms were forced to step in. Jails and prisons became the default facilities for mental illness. These were never meant to be therapeutic environments—they were built for containment, not care.

Today, more than *2 million people with mental illness are booked into jails each year.* Many are arrested for nonviolent crimes associated with the symptoms of their untreated conditions—erratic behavior, paranoia, trespassing, loitering. We have made suffering into something punishable. We treat psychosis as deviance. We equate mental disorganization with threat.

When law enforcement becomes the default responder to mental health crises, tragedy often follows. Officers are not trained mental health professionals. Most are not equipped to de-escalate psychiatric episodes safely. Even with the growth of Crisis Intervention Team (CIT) programs, far too many families still report harm where they asked for help. This shift has turned mental illness into a public safety issue rather than a public health one.

This systemic failure doesn't just traumatize individuals—it devastates families. It creates a cycle of fear: if we seek help, will our loved one be harmed? If we stay silent, will things get worse?

What happens *after* the arrest?

People with mental illness in jails are less likely to receive appropriate care, more likely to be placed in solitary confinement 23 out of 24 hours a day, and far more likely to be abused or retraumatized. Upon release, most leave without medication, a care plan, or a place to go—only to repeat the cycle again.

> We are not criminalizing danger.
> We are criminalizing distress.
> We are criminalizing suffering.

Every time we do, we reinforce a system that was built to contain, not to heal.

The Disconnect Between Treatment, Housing, Law Enforcement, and Long-Term Care

If someone you love with a serious mental illness ever makes it to treatment, you may breathe a sigh of relief—briefly. But for many families, that's just the beginning of another exhausting, broken cycle.

Stabilized? Maybe.

Discharged? Almost certainly.

Supported after? Rarely.

Our systems—mental health care, housing, law enforcement, social services—were never designed to work together. They speak different languages, operate under conflicting goals, and rarely share data or coordinate care. A clinician can stabilize someone for 72 hours, but if there's no supportive housing or long-term treatment plan, that "stabilization" is a Band-Aid on a gaping wound.

Police may respond to a 911 call involving a mental health crisis, very often repeatedly to the same address for the same individual in crisis, but often lack the tools or training to de-escalate safely. And when jails become the de facto detox or holding tank for the mentally ill, we reinforce a pipeline that is both inhumane and ineffective.

Without integrated care—housing, therapy, case management, medication monitoring, peer support—stabilization is a temporary reprieve. It's not recovery; it's a pause before the next fall.

Our systems weren't built to talk to each other.

Mental health providers often aren't able to coordinate with housing authorities.

Police departments don't have access to crisis team backups in every city.

Jails discharge without wraparound planning.

Clinics operate on schedules that don't match the urgency of crisis.

So what happens?

Someone is released from a short-term psychiatric hold. There's no housing bed available. Their name is added to a months-long waitlist for therapy. They miss a follow-up appointment, and medication runs out. Symptoms return. The cycle restarts—now with more trauma layered on top.

This is the illusion of care. It looks like treatment, but without follow-through, it's only

containment. And don't mention the revolving door of turnover in clinicians that
causes another layer of issues.

We call it a "system," but in reality, it's a collec-
tion of isolated responses—none of which
communicate, none of which are designed for
sustained healing.

INTRODUCTION TO SYSTEMS FAILURE

When families say the system is broken, it's a
cry of pain. But the deeper truth is more sober-
ing: the system isn't broken—*it was never whole
to begin with.*

We were handed fragments:

> A Medicaid application here.
> An overworked case manager there.
> A 15-minute evaluation.
> A discharge paper.
> A police welfare check.

This isn't a system. It's triage in perpetuity.

The public institutions meant to care for our
most vulnerable are trapped in a loop of short-
term fixes. Policies prioritize liability over hu-
manity. Funding is reactive instead of preventa-

tive. Services exist in silos, and people fall between them—hard.

This isn't about individual failure—it's systemic neglect. And the more we treat mental illness as a series of isolated episodes rather than a chronic, complex condition deserving of integrated, compassionate care, the more we perpetuate trauma.

And families? We are expected to navigate it all. To advocate, coordinate, supervise, and survive. To stay calm in emergencies, learn legal codes, find beds, and keep hope alive. *But hope without help becomes heartbreak.*

Until we recognize mental illness as a long-term, complex, and deeply human challenge—one that requires compassion, collaboration, and continuity—we will continue to retraumatize those we claim to serve.

This isn't just a policy failure.

It is a moral failure.

And it is long past time to build a system that heals.

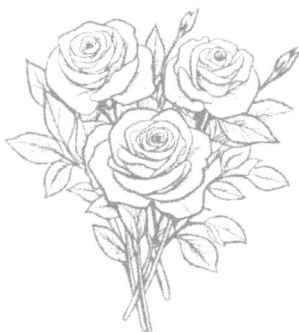

Above all else, guard your heart, for everything flows from it.

Proverbs 4:23

LESSON 2
No One Told Me How to Speak the Language

One of the most disorienting and isolating aspects of navigating the mental health system is that it has its own language—one that most of us never learned, and no one is offering to teach. The first time you sit across from a clinician who casually drops acronyms or diagnoses without explanation, or a caseworker who references statutes as if you've memorized the legal code, it hits you: you're in a system where everyone seems to speak a foreign dialect, and you're expected to translate in real time.

There is no welcome packet.

No orientation manual.

No glossary at intake.

No trauma-informed tour guide.

Instead, you're thrown into the deep end of a fragmented, high-stakes world of policies, paperwork, and procedures—and somehow, you're supposed to become fluent overnight.

And if you don't?

Your loved one can suffer—or worse, be lost entirely in the gaps.

NO CONTINUITY, NO HUB, NO INTERPRETER

There is no centralized hub in the mental health system—no unified agency that oversees care, communication, or continuity. Each door you walk through leads to a separate department, often with its own jargon, its own rules, and its own way of documenting information. The ER doesn't communicate with the outpatient psychiatrist. The case manager doesn't loop in the housing navigator. The judge may never read the hospital report. The mobile crisis team you begged for last week might not have jurisdiction today, or worse may not even still exist due to lack of funding.

So what happens?

You become the hub.

The translator.

The coordinator.

The historian.

You're asked to retell your loved one's story—again and again and again—because systems don't talk to each other, and providers don't always listen to families. Worse, when you can't "speak the language" fluently—when you pause, hesitate, or ask for clarification—you're often treated as if you're part of the problem. You're told you're confused. Or too emotional. Or "noncompliant." The burden of communication is placed squarely on you, the caregiver, regardless of your background, trauma load, or access to support.

This isn't just frustrating. It's dangerous.

The Terms No One Taught You

Some terms are clinical. Some are legal. Some are bureaucratic shorthand. But none of them are typically explained. And many have life-altering consequences. For example:

• **5150 (California)**: An involuntary psychiatric hold for individuals deemed a danger to self or others or gravely disabled. Other states have different names. For example, in Kentucky the term is 202A or 202B and in Ohio it's referred to as "Pink Slipping". Rarely is the process clearly outlined for families.

• **LPS Conservatorship**: A legal designation under California law that assigns someone the right to make decisions on behalf of a person with serious mental illness. Other states may call it guardianship, commitment, or protective services.

• **IEP**: Individualized Education Program—essential for children with disabilities in public schools, but often misunderstood or mis-applied.

• **DSM (Diagnostic and Statistical Manual of Mental Disorders)**: The standard classification system used to diagnose psychiatric conditions. Currently in its 5th edition (DSM-5-TR).

• **ACT Team (Assertive Community Treatment)**: A multidisciplinary team providing wraparound, in-community support for individuals with high psychiatric needs. Many families have never even heard of this option.

• **SMI & SPMI (Serious Mental Illness; Serious and Persistent Mental Illness)**: A legal and clinical classification that affects eligibility for services—but the criteria for qualifying are often unclear or inconsistently applied.

• **AOT (Assisted Outpatient Treatment)**: The practice of providing community-based mental health treatment under civil court commitment, as a means of: (1) motivating an adult with mental illness who struggles with voluntary treatment adherence to engage fully with their treatment plan; and (2) focusing the attention of treatment providers on the need to work diligently to keep the person engaged in effective treatment.

• **Medical Release:** A Medical Release is a legal document that authorizes the disclosure of an individual's protected health information (PHI) from a healthcare provider, hospital, or other medical entity to a specified third party, such as another healthcare provider, family member, legal representative, or organization. It is typically used to comply with privacy laws, such as the Health Insurance Portability and Accountability Act (HIPAA) in the United States, which restricts the sharing of medical information without patient consent.

• **Mental Incompetency:** Refers to a legal determination that an individual lacks the mental ability to make informed decisions about specific aspects of their life, such as financial matters, healthcare, or legal affairs. It is typically a formal ruling made by a court or legal authority.

• **Capacity:** Refers to an individual's ability to understand, process, and make informed decisions about specific situations or tasks at a given time. It is typically assessed in a medical or clinical context rather than a legal one.

By the time you figure out what half of these terms mean, your loved one may have already cycled through three placements, lost housing, or ended up in jail. That's the cost of a language barrier. And it's a barrier most families face with no translator and no training.

The Acronym Avalanche: How Language Obscures Power

Every field has jargon, but in mental health, language isn't just technical—it's a gatekeeper. It creates an invisible wall between those who are "in the know" and those who aren't. And that wall can keep families from accessing life-saving services.

Language is not neutral.

It is a form of power.

And families—especially those without legal training, clinical background, or native English proficiency—are often left powerless in the very moments they need the most support.

Mental Illness vs. Mental Health vs. Behavioral Health

Let's demystify a few core terms that are often conflated:

- **Mental Illness** refers to diagnosable psychiatric conditions like schizophrenia, bipolar disorder, or PTSD. These are typically long-term and may require medical treatment, therapy, and community support.

- **Mental Health** is a broader concept that encompasses emotional wellness, resilience, and coping mechanisms. Everyone has mental health, just like everyone has physical health—but not everyone has a mental illness.

- **Behavioral Health** is a term frequently used in health systems to encompass both mental health and substance use treatment. In many settings, behavioral health departments handle everything from addiction recovery to outpatient counseling to psychiatric medication management.

These distinctions matter. They affect insurance coverage, provider qualifications, treatment options, and access to resources. Misunderstanding these terms can lead to inappropriate referrals, denied care, or unnecessary delays.

The Trauma of Not Knowing

What no one tells you is that simply *not knowing the language* can become its own form of trauma. You sit in meeting after meeting, hearing words you don't understand, watching professionals scribble in charts and nod to each other, while your gut screams that something is wrong—but you can't name it.

> You don't know what questions to ask.
> You don't know what rights you have.
> You don't know what options exist.
> You blame yourself for not knowing.

But it's not your fault.

The system wasn't designed to include you—it was designed to protect itself.

What Families Need

Families need more than pamphlets. We need:

• Plain language communication

• Interpreters and advocates trained in trauma-informed practices

• Glossaries and orientation at the point of entry

• Case managers who explain the why, not just the what

• Providers who listen, not just diagnose

When families understand the language, we can ask better questions. We can anticipate barriers. We can prepare for transitions. We can advocate effectively.

Most of all—we can stop being left out of conversations about the people we love.

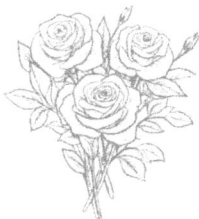

Then I heard the voice of the Lord saying,
"Whom shall I send? And who will go for us?"
And I said, 'Here am I. Send me!'

Isaiah 6:8

LESSON 3
NO ONE TOLD ME MY RIGHTS—OR MY CHILD'S

When someone you love is diagnosed with a serious mental illness—especially your child—you're pulled into a whirlwind of hospitals, evaluations, acronyms, and decisions you never imagined having to make. In the middle of this storm, you might look around and realize something terrifying: you don't actually know your rights. Or theirs. And no one is offering to tell you.

You're expected to navigate overlapping medical, legal, and educational systems as if you were trained to do so. But you're not. Most families don't get a guidebook until after the damage has been done—if ever.

This lesson is about reclaiming the power of information. It's about what every family needs to know on Day One (but often doesn't learn until Day 1,001). Because in a system that's reactive instead of proactive, the only way to make a difference is to know your rights, understand the laws, and prepare to fight for both.

WHAT FAMILIES NEED TO KNOW BUT AREN'T TOLD

We begin with the essentials: the legal and ethical rights that govern how information is shared, who can access care, and what decisions can (and cannot) be made without you.

HIPAA: THE LAW THAT BOTH PROTECTS AND BLOCKS

You've probably heard of HIPAA—the **Health Insurance Portability and Accountability Act**—but what does it really mean for families?

HIPAA was created to protect patient privacy, particularly in an age of digital records and insurance transitions. It is well-intentioned. But in practice, it often leaves families in the dark— especially when their adult loved one is in the middle of a mental health crisis.

Unless there's a signed medical release or your child is a minor, clinicians may be *prohibited* from speaking with you—even if your loved one is on a psychiatric hold or in acute distress.

You may find yourself desperately trying to pass on vital context—only to be told, "I can't confirm or deny that this patient is here."

One parent to another: Please—read the HIPAA law for yourself. Know what it actually says. Don't rely on assumptions or secondhand info. Your goal is the same as theirs: the safety and wellbeing of your loved one. Approach every conversation from that shared concern.

Tips for navigating HIPAA:

• **Ask about medical releases early and often.** Don't wait for a crisis.

• **Frame your communication as helpful.** ("Here's something I think might help in your assessment.")

• **Don't assume silence means hostility.** Sometimes providers are legally gagged. Keep offering support and information, even if you receive nothing back.

Patient Rights: Know Them Before You Need Them

Patients—yes, even those in psychiatric crisis—retain a host of legal rights. These may include:

- The **right to refuse treatment**, unless legally deemed incompetent.

- The **right to be informed** about their diagnosis and care options.

- The **right to access their own medical records.**

These rights matter—but they're not always easy to exercise or enforce. Many families discover them only *after* care has been denied, cut off, or mishandled.

Understanding these rights ahead of time allows you to speak with confidence, request documentation, and know when your loved one's autonomy is being violated—or when the system is acting within bounds.

Guardianship & Legal Authority

In some cases, families may need to seek **legal guardianship** or **conservatorship**—especially when an adult child is unable to make informed decisions due to severe mental illness.

This is not a quick or easy process. It involves legal filings, possible court appearances, and often resistance—from the system *and* from the loved one in question.

Still, for some families, guardianship is a necessary tool to:

• Ensure consistent access to medical updates.

• Authorize treatment when a person lacks capacity.

• Manage finances or living arrangements when stability is elusive.

Be aware: laws around guardianship vary by state, and success often depends on clear documentation and legal advocacy.

Advocacy: What It *Really* Looks Like

In theory, advocacy is simple: speak up on behalf of someone who can't speak for themselves. But in practice, advocacy is much more than raising your voice. It's:

• Learning a new system while grieving or panicking.

Asking the same question five times until you get a clear answer.

• Showing up, again and again, when the doors keep closing.

• Always looking for the next option, when it

feels like there are no more options, or at least none that you haven't tried.

• Sometimes it means doing the same things again that have already been tried. Keep trying.

Most importantly: it's about not giving up, even when you're exhausted.

To become an effective advocate, you must become a researcher, a record-keeper, a negotiator, and a networker. You'll learn quickly that the system won't hand you the tools—you'll have to build them yourself.

Advocacy Tips: Speak Up, Document, and Build a Village

Here are practical strategies every family advocate should know:

1. Speak Up

• Always remember: *you are the expert* on your child.
• Ask direct, specific questions: "What are the next steps?" "Who is the point of contact?" "Is there a treatment plan in writing?"
• Use respectful persistence. "I'm not trying to overstep, but I need to un-

derstand how this decision was made."

• Seek to understand, before being understood. This is accomplished best by listening carefully, then asking poignant questions.

2. Document Everything

• Create a dedicated journal, binder, or digital folder.
• Track dates, names, phone numbers, and summaries of every interaction.
• Keep copies of IEPs, psychological evaluations, discharge notes, letters from doctors, etc.
• Keep your own notes when official documents may not be available. Your notes may become very important documentation later.

Documentation is power. In meetings, legal disputes, or appeals, your records will be your strongest ally.

3. Build a Support Network

You are not alone. Connect with:

- **Parent mentors** who've been through it.
- **Disability and mental health rights organizations** (like NAMI, The Arc, Disability Rights Centers, Treatment Advocacy Center, Mental Health America).
- **Online communities**, local advocacy groups, and support networks.
- Seek out advocates who can coach you through appeals, IEP meetings, or court hearings.

The journey is too long to walk alone. Find people who can stand beside you—and offer you both resources and rest.

A Note on Emotional Advocacy

Your voice matters, but so does your *tone*. Advocacy isn't just about facts—it's about how you show up. You'll make more progress when you approach professionals as collaborators, not enemies. But that doesn't mean being passive. You can be firm and kind. Clear and compassionate. Relentless and respectful.

When the system sees you as informed, prepared, and united with others—you are no longer easy to dismiss.

Information *Is* Power

In this system, silence is the default. Information is withheld. Rights are buried in fine print. And the burden of understanding falls on the very people least equipped to carry it—families in pain, in panic, in crisis.

But the more you learn, the stronger you become. The more you speak up, the more others will listen. And the more you demand transparency, the closer we move to a system that truly supports the people it's meant to serve.

You are not just a parent, sibling, spouse, or friend. You are an advocate. And knowledge is your armor.

The more you become informed, the more you learn that you are not alone.

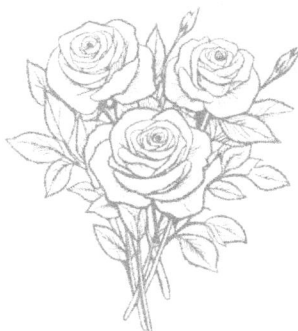

He has showed you, O God, what is good. And what does the Lord require of you? To act justly, and to love mercy and to walk humbly with your God.

Micah 6:8

LESSON 4
No One Told Me About the Waiting

No one tells you that one of the most grueling parts of navigating the mental health and disability system isn't the paperwork, the diagnoses, or the meetings—it's the waiting.

You wait for a phone call.
You wait for an appointment.
You wait for services to start, approvals to come through, medications to take effect.
You wait for your loved one's illness to improve; it can take so long sometimes to see.
And sometimes, you wait just to be believed.

One of the hardest nights of my life was spent sitting in a cramped emergency room with my child, both of us exhausted, scared, and confused. I thought this visit would finally bring answers, a clear path, maybe even a hospital bed. Instead, we were discharged with a stack of referral papers and a vague suggestion to "follow up with outpatient care." No timeline. No coordination. Just... wait.

That this broken moment *was* the system. And that from here, we'd have to fight—sometimes daily—for scraps of care while time slipped by and needs grew heavier.

Waiting isn't just about time. It's about the emotional erosion that happens when urgency meets a system that moves at the speed of molasses. It's about feeling powerless while trying to stay strong for someone who depends on you. It's about being expected to hold everything together, even as you watch it unravel.

HAVE A PLAN NOW—NOT LATER

Here's the hardest truth: the system rarely meets you where you are. You have to meet it head-on—with a plan, a binder, a backup list, and the tenacity of someone who refuses to be dismissed.

Waiting doesn't have to mean doing nothing. Preparation is your armor.

• **Know who you can call before a crisis happens.** Build a short list of trusted providers

—therapists, pediatricians, psychiatric nurse practitioners, case managers—people who return calls, listen well, and know your story.

• **Understand your insurance policy.** Know your coverage, your co-pays, what requires pre-approval, and how to file an appeal. Take notes when speaking to providers and ask for everything in writing.

• **Map your resources.** Look beyond the medical model. Are there local nonprofits offering respite care? Is there a faith community with a support ministry? Parent-led organizations? Family advocates at the school? Cast a wide net —you never know who might become a lifeline.

• **Create a Crisis Plan.** Don't wait until the next meltdown, shutdown, or emergency room visit to figure out what to do. Write it down. Include:

   ◦ Emergency contacts
   ◦ Medications, dosages, and providers
   ◦ Preferred hospital (if any)
   ◦ Documents to bring (guardianship papers, IEPs, diagnoses)
   ◦ What calms your child (this matters more than people realize)

Even if your plan gets interrupted or rerouted, having one is an act of power. It reminds you that you're not helpless—you're prepared.

THE EMOTIONAL WEIGHT OF WAITING

Waiting with uncertainty is one thing. Waiting while watching your child or loved one struggles, regresses, or loses hope—that's another. It can feel like being trapped in a loop you didn't choose and can't escape.

> You might feel guilt. Rage. Despair.
> You might question your instincts or wonder if you're "doing enough."
> You may start mourning the version of life you thought you'd have.

And through it all, the system just keeps... not calling.

This is why community matters. When no one else sees the urgency, other parents do. When professionals say, "just be patient," someone in your circle can say, "I know. Me too." These aren't small things. They're survival tools.

Tips for Surviving the Wait While Staying Resilient

Here are some of the things that have kept me afloat, and that I now offer to you—from one exhausted-but-still-holding-on parent to another:

1. Build a Support Network (and Use It)

Don't wait for permission to find your people. Join a Facebook group. Attend a support meeting, even virtually. Ask your child's school if they have parent mentors. The strongest advocates I've met were once scared and alone, just like you.

2. Practice Self-Care Without Guilt

Self-care doesn't mean spa days. It means deep breaths in the car before walking into an IEP meeting. It means giving yourself permission to cry in the laundry room. It means letting yourself watch a show or eat dinner in silence. You matter. Your mental health matters. You cannot pour from an empty cup.

3. Keep a Journal or Binder

Document everything. Every call you made. Every symptom you saw. Every time you were told "no" or "just wait." Over time, these notes will become your evidence, your advocacy tool, your timeline, your receipt of all the ways you've shown up.

4. Celebrate the Tiny Victories

That phone call you finally made? That email you sent? The fact that you got through another week without giving up? That counts. Celebrate it. You're climbing a mountain with little help and a heavy load—don't overlook how far you've come.

5. Remind Yourself That Waiting Doesn't Define You

You are not weak because you are waiting. You are not doing it wrong because the system is slow. The delay is not your fault. What *is* yours is your commitment. Your love. Your fight. And none of that is on pause.

From One Parent to Another: I don't have a magic fix for the brokenness we're forced to navigate. But I do know this: you are not alone. And you're not failing because your loved one's services are delayed, or because you cried in the car again today. That's not failure. That's what survival looks like in a system that doesn't move fast enough for the people who need it most.

So hold onto your hope. Keep your binder close. Build your village. And remember—this is the hard part, but not the whole story. There will be moments of progress, of laughter, of light. They may come slower than you want— but they do come.

You are doing more than waiting. You are enduring. You are preparing. You are showing up, every day, with love.

That is nothing short of heroic.

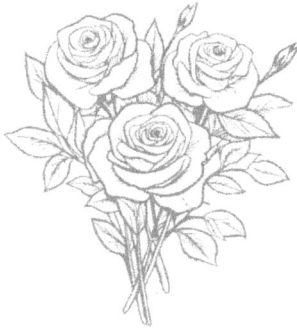

You will keep in perfect peace him whose mind is steadfast, because he trusts in you.

Isaiah 26:3

LESSON 5
NO ONE TOLD ME THE SYSTEM MIGHT BLAME ME...

One of the most painful and unexpected challenges families face—especially mothers and primary caregivers—is the shame and suspicion that can come with simply trying to seek help. No one prepared me for how isolating that experience would be. When your loved one is struggling—whether it's with mental health, neurodivergence, or disability—you expect professionals to offer support. But what happens when the questions they ask imply that *you* are the problem?

When I first voiced concerns about my child or loved one's behaviors, I was met not with validation, but with side glances, hesitations, and subtle skepticism. "Have you tried more structure?" "Are you consistent at home?" "Maybe they're just reacting to something in the environment." Each comment felt like a polite way of pointing the finger at me.

There's an unspoken accusation that floats through the system: *If your child is struggling, it must be because of something you did—or failed to do.* And when you're already running on empty, already questioning yourself, that kind of stigma doesn't just hurt—it carves into your confidence and self-worth.

EXCLUSION IN DISGUISE

The blame doesn't always sound like blame. Sometimes, it shows up in the form of exclusion. You might hear, "Maybe this environment just isn't the right fit," or "We don't have the staff to support those needs." Translation? *You're no longer welcome here.*

We've been asked to leave places—schools, camps, group events—because our child's behavior was misunderstood or inconvenient. Not disruptive. Not dangerous. Just different. And it was heartbreaking every time.

The places that should have embraced us became the very places that pushed us out. Over time, the impact of that exclusion becomes cumulative: fewer invitations, fewer friendships, fewer moments of feeling seen. It's not just your child who feels the sting of rejection—it's you too. You begin to wonder if your family will ever be fully accepted, or if you're destined to stay on the margins.

The Silent Toll on Mothers

As mothers, we carry an invisible backpack of responsibility. We absorb the appointments, the therapies, the advocacy, the logistics. But we also carry the emotional weight—the judgment from others, the inner questioning, the tears cried quietly behind closed doors.

I've sat in IEP meetings where professionals look to me to provide answers that I thought they should be providing to me, not the other way around. I've had to retell our story over and over, trying to receive the help we needed to save my son's life, trying to convince someone that I wasn't just an anxious mom blowing things out of proportion. That kind of emotional labor takes a toll.

It's no wonder so many of us experience burnout, anxiety, and depression. It's not just the demands of caregiving—it's the crushing burden of navigating a system that too often treats us with suspicion, or indifference, instead of support.

Rewriting the Narrative

Here's what I've learned: you do not have to carry that blame. You did not cause this. You are not alone.

Start by finding one person who sees you *without judgment.* A therapist, another parent, an advocate—someone who helps you remember your truth. Build your community around those who *get it*—not just intellectually, but emotionally.

Document everything. Not just to protect yourself (although that's part of it), but to remind yourself of your efforts, your intuition, and your unwavering love.

Most importantly: be kind to yourself. You are showing up every single day in a system that wasn't designed to support you. That in itself is heroic.

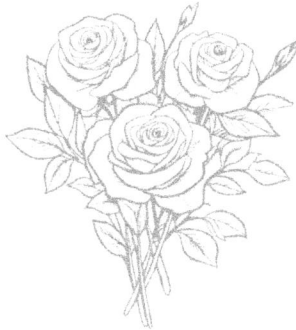

In his heart a man plans his course, but the Lord determines his steps.

Proverbs 16:9

LESSON 6
NO ONE TOLD ME THE SYSTEM MIGHT BE IMPOSSIBLE TO NAVIGATE

THE MAZE OF SERVICES, PAPERWORK, AND THE NEVER-ENDING WAIT

I thought once we received the correct diagnosis—or at least got someone to listen—things would start to fall into place. I believed the hardest part was behind us. What no one told me was that getting support wasn't a straight line. It was more like a maze or putting a puzzle together when the pieces keep changing.

In mental illness, especially in young people, it can often feel like the target is moving. That's because it is. It's not your imagination. Bodies grow and gain weight. Hormones change through puberty. Medications that once work, stop working.

Adding to those challenges, the system is a patchwork of agencies, acronyms, and applications. Mental health services live in one place. Educational supports in another. Insurance in yet another. Every doorway requires a different key—documentation, evaluations, proof of need, income statements, waitlists, and persistence. Endless persistence.

Sometimes I'd make it through one door, only to find out the next one was closed for now. Doctors leave service providers; new relationships must start all over. Providers discontinue services leaving gaping holes for help. Bills for treatment, even after insurance, mount up like mountains. It wasn't just frustrating. It was *devastating*—because the stakes were always so high. I wasn't chasing convenience; I was chasing survival. Safety. A lifeline for my child.

Mental health is the only area of health that individuals are expected… no, *required*, to fail (and keep failing) to receive the help they need. Try this. That didn't work. Try that. That didn't work. Years and years of trying, failing, trying, failing. Meanwhile your loved one gets sicker and sicker.

To illustrate, imagine being diagnosed with a rapidly progressing cancer at Stage 1, but instead of immediate, aggressive treatment, you're told to try basic interventions or wait and see. You're only offered the intensive, life-saving treatment appropriate for cancer's severity when it's reached Stage 4, when the disease has become far harder to control. This is the reality for many with severe mental illness: the treatment provided often doesn't match the condition's gravity.

Why must we watch our loved ones reach the equivalent of Stage 4 Cancer before they receive the help they need?

The Illusion of Help

One of the hardest things to grasp was that having a diagnosis didn't guarantee access to help. Even when professionals agreed something was wrong—even when I had binders of reports, years of documentation, and dozens of signatures—there was still no clear path forward.

Sometimes it felt like the system gave me just enough hope to keep me hanging on. I'd think, *Finally, we've made it through this part,* only to be told, "This program doesn't cover that," or "We no longer have funding," or "Try calling back in six months." I was told to wait, to call, to try again. Meanwhile, my child was struggling *right now.*

I often felt like I had to become an expert in everything: special education law, Medicaid waivers, therapeutic models, behavioral intervention plans. There was no map. No one to say, "Here's what you do next." It was all trial and error, with my child's well-being in the balance.

The Toll on Families and the Privilege of Access

And while navigating this system was hard for me—with a college degree, access to technology, and the time (barely) to research—it broke my heart to think of those who had less. What about the single mom working two jobs? The family with language barriers? The caregiver without reliable transportation or internet?

The truth is, the system isn't just hard to navigate—it's inequitable by design. Those who need the most help often face the most barriers. And the emotional cost of constantly being told "no," of starting over again and again, is something you carry in your bones.

No GPS for This Journey

There are times when I felt like the system was resisting our need. The authorities were resisting finding solutions. The professionals were resisting with diagnosis and meaningful support. My son was resisting me. Because after all, he didn't see himself as sick. It felt like resistance was on all sides. Resistance to what? Resistance to my son getting the help that he desparately needed-without any melodrama at all-the help he needed to stay alive.

But was the system really resisting me? No, not really. The system did what the system does.

I felt like I was failing. But now I know: *I wasn't failing. The system was failing me.*

What I Want You to Know

If you've ever felt like the help you need is just out of reach, or that you must be doing something wrong because the system makes no sense —you are not alone.

You're not imagining the confusion, the complexity, or the exhaustion. The system *is* broken, or more accurately, it was never built to effectively manage the mental health need, especially the need created after institutions were shuttered.

So here's what I want you to remember:

• **Your instincts are valid.** If you think your child needs help, you're right to keep pushing.

- **Find the guides.** Seek out advocates, parent mentors, or social workers who know the landscape. Don't try to do it all alone.

- **Take breaks.** You don't have to win every battle in a single day. Rest is part of resilience.

- **Document everything.** Emails, dates, conversations. These can be your compass—and your protection.

Most of all, be gentle with yourself. You are doing the impossible inside a system that often makes survival feel like a miracle. And still— you are here. You're showing up. You're trying.

That is not failure. That is love. That is bravery. That is the work of a fierce and determined parent navigating a path no one warned you about—and refusing to give up.

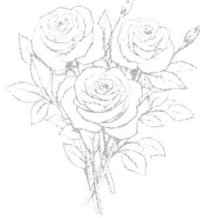

Finally brothers, whatever is true, whatever is noble, whatever is right, whatever is pure, whatever is lovely, whatever is admirable-if anything is excellent or praiseworthy-think about such things. Whatever you have learned or received or heard from me, or even seen in me-put into practice. And the God of peace will be with you.

Philippians 4:8

LESSON 7
NO ONE TOLD ME THAT CHANGE WAS POSSIBLE

FINDING POWER IN PERSISTENCE, AND PURPOSE IN THE FIGHT

For so long, I could have become so discouraged when change didn't come, or at least not fast enough. Why wouldn't I feel discouraged? Why wouldn't you?

When you're caught in the whirlwind of crisis and survival—navigating hospitalizations, courtrooms, emergency conversations with authorities, calls with law enforcement, or during long periods when the system saw my son as less than worthy of the help he needed —you begin to lose sight of anything beyond the next fire you have to put out. You learn how to live in urgency, not because you want to, but because the systems around you leave you no other choice.

Hope starts to feel like a luxury for other people—people with more resources, better connections, or a child who fits more neatly into the boxes the world understands. It's not that you stop believing in good things. It's that good things begin to feel like they were made for someone else.

But I've learned something that changed me: hope isn't a fantasy. It's a practice. A discipline. A strategy.

PLACE YOUR HOPE WHERE IT CAN DO SOMETHING

I no longer place my hope in the system doing the right thing on its own. That kind of passive hoping will leave you depleted, disillusioned, and quietly resentful. But I *do* place my hope in the people willing to show up *in* and *against* that system. Families. Caregivers. Advocates. Survivors. Professionals who choose compassion over red tape. Those who understand because they've been there.

That is where the shift begins.

Change doesn't always announce itself. It rarely arrives as sweeping reform in headlines or legislative bills. Most of the time, it sneaks in through back doors and side conversations. It looks like:

• A professional who finally says, "I believe you."

• When you finally see some improvement, no matter how small-to the services being made available or improvement in behaviors attributed to medication compliance.

• When someone says, I'm not supposed to do this, but I'm going to help you, because I see you are a Mom who loves her son and you are just trying to help him, when he can't help himself.

These changes might seem small to outsiders— but they're everything to the families impacted by them. And they stack. Like bricks in a wall. Like steps in a revolution.

Stories of Progress: The Power of One Step

Let me be clear: I've seen what one step can do. I've seen the road that is paved by staying the course-one step at a time.

I've seen a single testimony change a lawmaker's perspective. I've watched mothers and fathers who were once overlooked become local leaders, running support networks, influencing policy, building programs from scratch. I've seen Statehouses and Congressional phone lines flooded with calls demanding change.

I've witnessed caregivers—*exhausted but not defeated*—build coalitions out of pain. I've seen children once written off by the system bloom in spaces where they were finally seen.

These moments didn't come from power. They came from *persistence.* From families who refused to give up. From people who were tired of feeling voiceless and decided to speak anyway.

That's what makes the biggest difference. Not perfection. Not permission. Just the decision to begin.

You Can Be Part of the Movement

Advocacy can feel intimidating. Politics can feel far away. Systems can seem too big to move. But everything changes when we remember that systems are made of people—and people can change.

You don't have to know everything. You don't have to do it all. You just have to start.

Here are a few real, tangible ways to begin:

- **Educate yourself.** Learn the laws. Learn your rights. Knowledge is armor and fuel.

- **Share your story.** In a meeting. On social media. At a rally. With your neighbor. Every story chips away at stigma.

- **Build bridges.** Invite your local officials to your events. Follow up with emails. Make them see the lives behind the numbers. Talk to your legislatures. Educate them.

Join others. Plug into local and national advocacy groups. Volunteer. Amplify. Collaborate.

- **Vote.** Local elections matter. Judges matter. School boards matter. Your vote is a tool— use it.

You don't need a title to make a difference. You just need your story, and the courage to offer it.

What I'm Doing—and How You Can Join Me

I used to think my only option was survival. That if I could just keep my head down, stay under the radar, and keep my child safe, that was the win.

But surviving is not the same as living. And silence doesn't protect us—it isolates us.

Now, I speak up.

I sit on boards and commissions—not because I have all the answers, but because I bring the *lived* answers. I advocate not because I was trained to, but because I had no other choice. I have become so passionate about advocating that if I didn't do it, I would shrivel up and cease to exist.

I've created programs, published books, launched initiatives, led organizations, and partnered with people who want to make this world more livable for families like mine—and yours.

And I'm still learning. Still fighting. Still believing.

Most of all: I'm still *hoping*.

I'm inviting you to do the same.

Pick one thing.

Make the call. Send the email. Ask the question. Show up.

Let that be the beginning of *your* change story.

Because no one told us change was possible.

But it is.

And it starts with us.

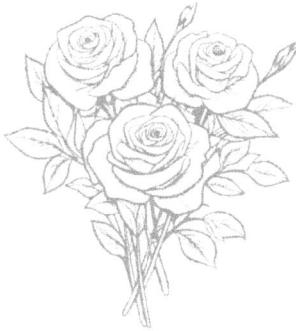

*We also rejoice in our sufferings, because we
know that suffering produces perseverance;
perseverance, character; and character, hope.
And hope, does not disappoint us, because God
has poured out his love into our hearts by the
Holy Spirit, whom he has given us.*

Romans 5:3-5

One Mother's Wait

By Wendy Jennings

I waited in a hospital room for four long weeks on his arrival.

I waited to hear him take his first breath and cry.

I waited four weeks to hold him in my arms.

I waited I waited six long weeks to take him home.

I waited fifteen months for him to take his first steps.

I waited a year and a half for him to come off the apnea monitor.

I waited for the right teacher, the right school, the right administrator to treat him with kindness and respect when he didn't check all the boxes.

I waited for the numerous doctors and specialists to tell me what was wrong instead of what was right with my son.

I waited fourteen years for ...a diagnosis of bipolar.

I waited for the right medications to "work".

I waited for the day he could graduate from high school.

I waited for the right job that he could perform work with the right supervisor that would understand ADHD, Asperger, Bi-Polar.

I waited while he had a psychotic break after being introduced to meth while on the job.

I waited numerous times while he was in recovery programs, in patient units, jail and prison.

I waited for him to come home and maintain sobriety.

I now wait for him to do the simple things in life like maintain his balance while walking, his memory, to return, and have a typical life at age 33.

Instead ...

I wait for the specialists to come up with answers after surgery for the head injuries he received in prison.

I wait for my Son to have a "normal" day in his life and I will continue to wait and advocate for him as long as it takes.

Afterword

This road is long and often lonely. But loneliness doesn't mean you're lost. It just means the world hasn't caught up to your reality yet.

You are not alone—and you were never meant to be. So let this be the moment you decide not to wait for permission.

You are allowed to hope.
You are allowed to demand better.
You are allowed to take up space in systems that would rather forget you.
You are not invisible.
Your voice is a light.

And together—we build the path forward.

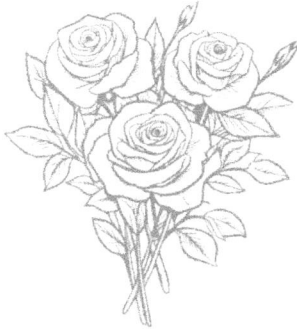

Be still and know that I am God.

~ Psalms 46:10a

ABOUT THE AUTHOR

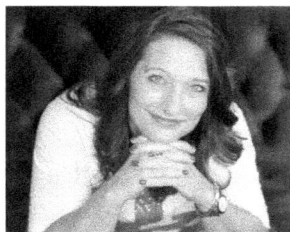

Kimberly A. Bowman is a seasoned nonprofit executive, mental health advocate, and public policy strategist with over two decades of experience leading transformational change at the intersection of behavioral health and the justice system. She has served as Executive Director of local National Alliance on Mental Illness (NAMI) chapter, Director of Employee Relations at a state psychiatric hospital, an Executive Director at a national human services organization in the Intellectual and Developmental Disability space—bringing mission-driven leadership to the forefront of her career.

Her passion for reform is deeply personal. As the mother of an adult son living with a severe and persistent mental health diagnosis, Kimberly has spent more than 45 years navigating the complexities of the mental health system. This lived experience has shaped her unshakable commitment to building a more compassionate, coordinated, and effective system of care. She understands firsthand the heartbreaking gaps in services, the fragmentation of care, the criminalization of mental illness, and the devastating cycles of justice involvement and homelessness. These challenges have fueled her determination to find real, scalable solutions that bring healing—not just to individuals in crisis, but to the families and communities that love and support them.

Kimberly is actively involved in Crisis Intervention Training (CIT) for law enforcement and is passionate about bridging the gap between public safety and behavioral health. As a certified pet therapy volunteer, she finds great joy in providing comfort and support to first responders, law enforcement officers, and firefighters. She lives in Michigan with her very supportive husband and her loyal therapy dog and continues to write, speak, and lead efforts that advance dignity, recovery, and justice for all.

www.ingramcontent.com/pod-product-compliance
Lightning Source LLC
Chambersburg PA
CBHW060254030426
42335CB00014B/1698